Relieve Stress With this Ancient Secret

A Psychiatrist Shows You How

Karen Ritchie, M.D.

ISBN: 978-1-62747-407-8
eBook ISBN: 978-1-62747-016-2

Dedication

For Olga, and all the other Olgas out there

Disclaimer

Nothing in this book is intended to diagnose or treat any medical illness. If you have a problem that requires professional attention, please contact your health care provider. If you have had major trauma, please work with a trained therapist. If you have suicidal thoughts, please get help immediately.

Contents

Prologue ix

Chapter 1 – The Ancient Secret 1

Chapter 2 – Why Should I Be Interested in the Ancient Secret?......... 5

Chapter 3 – The EFT Process 9

Chapter 4 – Acupuncture Comes to the United States...................... 19

Chapter 5 – If This Is So Great, Why Have I Never Heard of It? 23

Chapter 6 – More About EFT 29

Chapter 7 – I'm Stressed Now 31

Chapter 8 – I'm Always Stressed.. 33

Chapter 9 – What Do I Say? 41

Chapter 10 – What if it Doesn't Work? 47

Chapter 11 – What Is the Downside? 53

Chapter 12 – And Finally 59

Acknowledgements... 63

Prologue

Olga was having trouble lying still on the hospital cart. The nurse was trying to take her vital signs, but Olga was so panicked that she couldn't stand having anyone touch her, especially someone she didn't know. She did let her sister hold her hand and rub her arm, but that was all she could tolerate, and it didn't help much.

Her sister had taken her to the emergency room at the Veterans Administration hospital after she had called, and scolded her for not calling sooner. Olga had panic attacks often, sometimes daily, but this was one of the worst. She feared she was having a heart attack, or dying, or both.

The doctor came quickly, at the insistence of the nurse. He noted that Olga had been seen earlier that day in the mental health clinic but was not given any medications. He gave her intravenous medication to calm her down, which made her sleepy. He sent her home with a bottle of tablets, which she never took.

I was the psychiatrist she had seen earlier that day, and I was forbidden to help her. And it is partly because of Olga that you have this book.

Sadly, this is a true story, although the veteran's name is not Olga and I have changed some of the details. I was working in the clinic Olga visited, which treated veterans with post-traumatic stress disorder. I had been teaching other veterans the Ancient Secret that I discuss in this book. Many of the veterans had very good results and were encouraging their friends and colleagues to use it also. They invited me to their therapy groups and classes to teach the technique to others. But the supervisor ordered me to stop, and banned the technique from being used in the clinic.

Olga had tried taking medication in the past, but she found it too sedating and refused to try it again. She was working, though only with great effort on her part, and was afraid she would lose her job if she was too drowsy. She had been offered psychotherapy, but had difficulty getting off work to make it to her appointments. However, her symptoms were so severe that she could not benefit from any of the few therapy techniques that the VA promotes.

There was little I could do. I could have shown her the Ancient Secret despite the fact that I was forbidden to do so. In the end, I decided to obey the command and not teach it to her. But I will not be silent. I am writing this book for Olga and the other Olgas out there. I don't want this technique to be a secret any more.

Chapter 1
The Ancient Secret

The Ancient Secret is that you are more than your physical body, more than your muscles and bones, more than the parts you can touch and measure and see under a microscope. Medicine has treatment for the body, the nerves, the skin and the chemistry. But there is also treatment for the energy system within the body.

Acupuncture, and its many modern variations, use the Ancient Secret. Acupuncture is a part of traditional Chinese medicine. It has been in the United States for as long as there have been Chinese living in the US, but it was not known about widely until an article written in the *New York Times* in 1971 by James Reston. The technique became popular among Americans and continues to be widely available to this day.

One version of the Ancient Secret is called Emotional Freedom Technique, or EFT, which was developed from an earlier technique called TFT. Both are a form of acupuncture that you can do yourself without needles. I have been teaching EFT to people for many years, and I can tell you that it is very effective for stress.

It doesn't work every time – nothing does. But it often helps, and sometimes it is life-changing. For this technique, instead of putting needles in the acupuncture points, you simply tap on specific points where the energy flows. The basic procedure takes five minutes to learn, although there are many tricks and techniques to make it more effective. In this book I will show you how to use it for yourself, and tell you some stories of how it has helped other people.

Some people get results with a very simple version of EFT. A few years ago I was working in a clinic for women veterans, most of whom had post-traumatic stress disorder. I was teaching the full version of EFT to anyone who was interested. But many of the veterans in this clinic had relief from stress with simply tapping on one point – the thumb point on the chart below.

I will describe the tapping points in more detail in a later chapter. But to get started with EFT, and try it for yourself, you might try tapping on the points on the chart. Many people have relief from stress from tapping on just one point – the thumb or collarbone points are commonly effective.

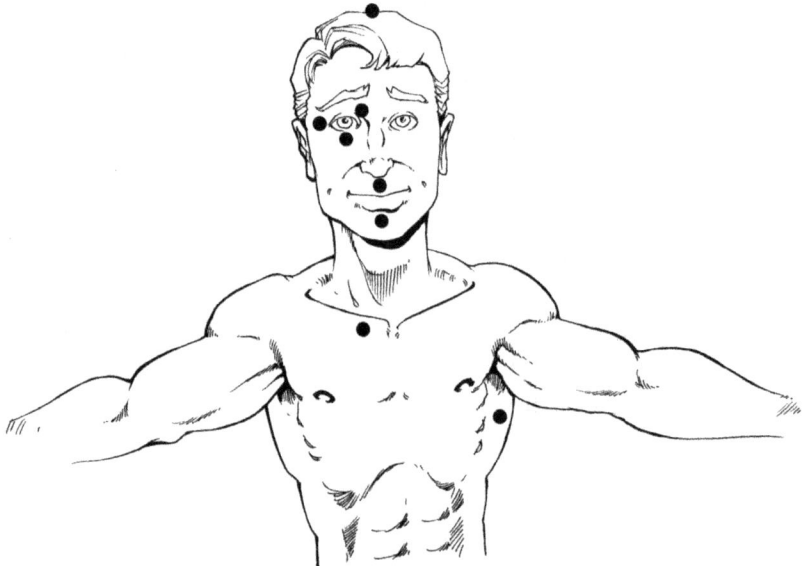

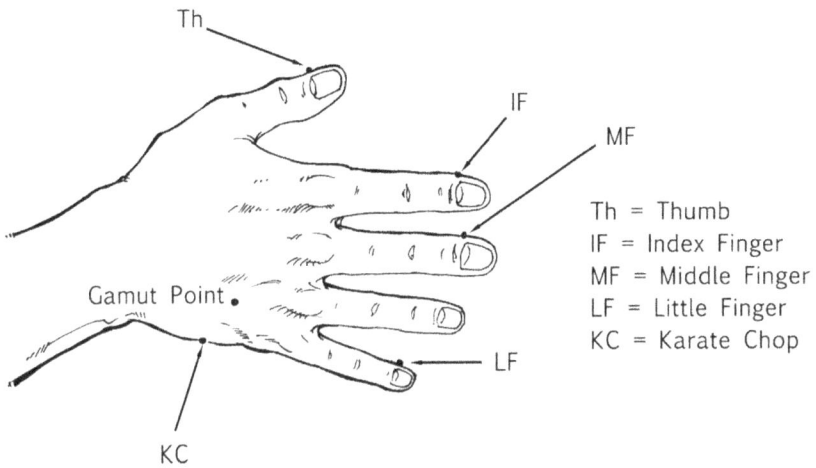

Th = Thumb
IF = Index Finger
MF = Middle Finger
LF = Little Finger
KC = Karate Chop

In Chinese medicine, the health of the body is considered to be maintained by the body's energy, called qi (pronounced chee). When this energy is out of balance or the flow is blocked, illness is the result.

This energy flows in pipelines, or meridians. You can find many diagrams on the internet that show where these meridians are located on the body. Acupuncture works on some of these points that are near the skin. (If you are interested in trying this out yourself, you can get an acupuncture point finder that will buzz or beep when you place it on one of these points. They can be found online.)

Acupuncture stimulates these meridian points by pressure, tapping, or by inserting needles. The theory is that this corrects the imbalance or blockage in the energy.

This technique is, indeed, ancient. The first known written record of acupuncture is in the oldest known medical textbook in the world, Huang Di Nei Jing (Yellow Emperor's Classic of Internal Medicine) which is dated at 4,700 years old and attributed to Shen Nung, the father of Chinese medicine.

Although acupuncture was thought to originate in China 4700 years ago, it may be even older, as evidenced by Ötzi, or the Ice Man, Europe's oldest natural mummy. He was found in September, 1991 in the Ötztal Alps, on the border between Austria and Italy, and is currently displayed in the South Tyrol Museum of Archaeology in Bolzano, South Tyrol, Italy. He lived around 3300 BC, which was before the Chinese Yellow Emperor's book.

Ötzi has over fifty tattoos in the form of groups of lines and crosses that are placed on skin acupuncture lines. He also was found to have physical problems that correspond to those meridians, leading to the assumption that the tattoos were placed as guides for acupuncture or acupressure.

Chapter 2
Why Should I Be Interested
in the Ancient Secret?

My friend had a lifelong fear of flying. She would panic whenever she had to get on an airplane, which she had to do on a regular basis. She tried medication and various relaxation techniques without results. I offered to show her EFT, but she was not interested. Eventually she decided to take a course on fear of flying offered by an airline. She paid the airline $500 for the class. Guess what they taught her? That's right. Tapping.

Susan Whitmire tells this story:

"My daughter-in-law introduced me to tapping, and she used it to overcome my issues with fresh peaches – peach fuzz. The kids used to chase me around with a peach, and you would have thought it was a tarantula or something. Now I can touch peaches and peel peaches, but I'm still not crazy about biting into one. So, I was in my fifties before fresh peaches were okay. All due to tapping. Proves it works for a lot of things."

What would you do if you weren't so stressed? Who would you be? What is the opposite of stress? The answer might be different for everyone.

Is your goal to be calm, or relaxed, or eager? Having fun? Being loving? Being productive? What would change for you if you could reduce your anxiety? What would you do differently?

You may feel stress around any number of issues. Work is a common source of tension. Do you dread going to work? Hate your job? If you're in a job that is unhealthy for you and you need to find a way out, reducing your stress level may help bring clarity and courage to make a move.

Do you like your job, but face a day full of obstacles to doing what you're supposed to do? I hear this frequently: "If only they would leave me alone and just let me do my job." Or is there just too much to do at work, and you can never get it all done? Does work creep into your unpaid personal time?

Financial stress is another common problem. Do you struggle to pay bills? Worry about money frequently? Worry about saving for retirement vs. today's needs?

Parenting is stressful under the best of conditions. You love your children and you know what kind of parent you want to be, but it is hard to measure up to our concept of the ideal parent. And/or you may be faced with aging parents and the many problems that brings.

A common cause of stress is problems in relationships, whether at home, at work, or with friends. In addition, the reverse is true. When you feel stressed, this is likely to cause more problems in your relationships. Many people find that when they are tense they keep more distance from others. You may find that your relationships are closer and more authentic when you are more relaxed. If you can reduce stress you may be able to be a better parent, spouse or employee.

Many of us are in situations where we must deal with unreasonable people or unreasonable conditions. There are likely people in your life that you really shouldn't have to deal with, but – there they are.

You may be like many people who feel overwhelmed, too busy, with not enough time or energy or money for everything in your life. You may feel that it's all too much, but you can't give up any of the pieces.

Some feel stressed but can't pinpoint a reason. If this happens to you, it is hard to fix because there is no apparent cause. You may be one who gets anxious and takes it out on those around you. Some have irrational fears – and justify them as being reasonable when they know they're not – and then feel guilty afterwards.

When you're stressed, you may feel alone, as if nobody else has this problem. Feeling isolated and alone is itself a source of stress. And yet, many of us are not honest enough to share our worries and problems with others. Alternately, you may see that everyone around you has the same problem you have, and conclude that it can't be solved.

Maybe your life doesn't fit who you are. Do you feel you're in the wrong place, that you need to be different, but life won't let you change and has you in a box? Is your life wearing you down and not letting you be the real you?

It's hard to get through life without having something traumatic happen to you. Many of us have old trauma that stays active, continuing to affect us. Please note: if you have a Big-T Trauma that is continuing to be a problem, consider seeing a therapist rather than trying to address it by yourself. But for other, small-t traumatic events, you may find the Ancient Secret helpful in reducing its impact on your life.

Chronic stress has well-documented effects on health conditions. If you reduce your stress, you may discover that you feel healthier. In addition, you may be more likely to do things that are within your control to improve your health, such as a better diet or more exercise.

The process in this book can help with both outside stress and inside stress. Outside stressors are the things we encounter in our life, such as difficult bosses, balky or whining children, an increase in rent, blizzards, all the big and small things that make life more difficult. We may or may not be able to change outside stressors, but we are always more effective when we're not tied up in knots.

Inside stress is the total of our worries, fears, disappointments, unpleasant memories, and the like. Inside stress can keep us small, keep us from growing.

Ironically, outside stress, when it is not overwhelming, can actually stimulate growth. Perhaps you have heard the story of the butterfly:

A man found a cocoon of a butterfly. One day, a small opening appeared. He sat and watched the butterfly for several hours as it struggled to squeeze its body through the tiny hole. Then it stopped, as if it couldn't go further.

So the man decided to help the butterfly. He took a pair of scissors and snipped off the remaining bits of cocoon. The butterfly emerged easily, but it had a swollen body and shriveled wings.

The man continued to watch it, expecting that any minute the wings would enlarge and expand enough to support the body. Neither happened! In fact, the butterfly spent the rest of its life crawling around. It was never able to fly.

What the man in his kindness and haste did not understand was that the restricting cocoon, and the struggle required by the butterfly to get through the opening, were necessary to force the fluid from the butterfly's body into its wings so that it would be able to fly.

Sometimes struggles are exactly what we need in our lives. Going through life with no obstacles would cripple us. We will not be as strong as we could have been – and we ourselves would never be able to fly. (Author unknown)

So a certain amount of stress can be like childbirth – difficult and painful at the time but productive – in this case, contributing to maturity and wisdom. On the other hand, too much stress can be overpowering and keep us from growing. Olga's panic attacks prevented her from doing anything, and they certainly were not helpful to her life in the long run.

Stress can keep us from growing to our full potential. We all have an area where we are comfortable, where we feel safe. But with less stress you can step out of your comfort zone. You can venture out more, get out more, live in a bigger world.

When you're less stressed, you may be willing to try new things. You are free to be more creative, to create better life conditions. You are likely to be more productive, as you are not spending energy on fears.

Many people get into a habit of feeling powerless over negative feelings. But with the process in this book, you have more control than you thought you did. You will have less need to control everything, but you will have more control over your life and your feelings. If you are worrying less, you have more ability to change what you don't like. You have an increased ability to see opportunities where you once saw problems or obstacles, and to have the optimism to take advantage of them. You can view your options more clearly when you are relaxed.

Do you feel you have a purpose in life? If so, it is probably not to stay home and stay safe. When you reduce stress you are more able to get out, move out, reach out, and follow your purpose.

And finally, if you reduce stress you will be able to relax, enjoy life more, and feel better. Do you need another reason?

Chapter 3
The EFT Process

A female veteran we'll call Barbara was being seen for post-traumatic stress disorder by my colleague, Joan Collins. She had had an experience thirty-five years earlier in which she was sexually assaulted by a group of men. She was now having flashbacks, with memory of the experience.

She had outpatient surgery, and in the recovery room, when she was regaining consciousness but not yet fully conscious, she had a panic attack. Although she needed another surgical procedure, the surgeon was unwilling to operate until the mental health service could assure him that she would not have another panic attack in the recovery room. In this case, time was of the essence, as she needed the second surgery as soon as possible. I was asked by Joan to provide EFT, as it works much faster than other forms of treatment.

At the first session, Barbara reviewed her history with Joan and me. I demonstrated how tapping works, and we addressed her current anxiety. After this session, Barbara used the tapping regularly to deal with her anxiety. The anxiety was reduced so much that family members began to ask her what was causing such a change in her.

During the second EFT session, she recovered a memory of the decades-old attack. She suddenly remembered that her attackers wore bandanas. She realized that when she was half-awake in the recovery room after surgery, and all the staff were wearing surgical masks, she had a flashback of the assault. This time, she asked the surgeon and nurses to take off their masks before speaking to her in the recovery room. The second surgery was done without incident, and without panic attacks.

The Process

Don't worry too much about getting it exactly right. There is more than one way to do the tapping. My colleague Cyndy White and I were reminded of this once when we were teaching tapping to veterans. In the first session of our class we would demonstrate the procedure, with a second session for answering questions and showing some additional options. One veteran, we'll call him Howard, came back the second week and reported great results with tapping. As he showed us how he was doing it, we could see that he was doing it very differently than we had demonstrated – he was doing several things that we had suggested he not do. In fact, he was doing it "incorrectly," and yet he was getting more symptom relief than anyone else in the class. I share Howard's story to demonstrate that this is a very forgiving process. It's hard to do it wrong.

Different people do it differently. In fact, Cyndy and I each use a slightly different method. We taught it to the group, each using our own technique, to make the point that there is more than one way to do tapping "correctly." If you look at videos online, and there are many, you will see a number of variations of the basic process. If it works, you are doing it right. If it doesn't work, try a different approach.

The first thing you do is to identify your goal. What do you want to accomplish with tapping? You give the problem a name. In your own words, say what the problem is that you want to address. So you may say "anxiety" or "this stress."

You may want to keep this part simple, with one or two words. So you could say "I am stressed," or "I'm always jumpy." Or you could give a more in-depth description – "I'm worried that I can't pay the bills this month." Either is fine – do what is comfortable for you.

You could state the problem in general terms, "I feel terrible." Or you could describe the problem in detail, "My boss just said that she doesn't like my proposal and I spent days on it. I'm so upset."

You want to answer the question, What do you want to be different? Why are you doing this? What do you want to get rid of?

Don't overthink this part – just say the obvious. Don't make it too hard or too elaborate. Your words don't have to be perfect. This process works on what you are thinking, and the words are just a way of focusing your thinking onto the problem. Otherwise you might get distracted into thinking about the weather, noises outside the room, or what you're going to have for dinner.

Now you measure how stressed you're feeling right now. This is called a SUDS, Subjective Units of Distress. It is similar to the rating scale used in healthcare for rating your pain, where the worst pain is a ten and no pain is a zero. You measure how stressed you are feeling on a scale of zero to ten, where ten is the most stressed you've ever felt and zero is the best you've ever felt. This doesn't have to be perfect. You just want to get a general idea of where your stress is right now so you can keep track of whether, and how far, it decreases with the tapping process. You may want to write down the SUDS number, or just remember it.

Setup

For the setup, you tap on the karate chop point, which is the fleshy area on the side of the hand between the little finger and the wrist. You want to state the problem, and then "I'm open to the possibility that I could feel better." So, some examples of setup statements would be:

"Even though I'm stressed right now, I'm open to the possibility that I could feel better."

"Even though I'm worried about these bills, I'm open to the possibility that I could relax."

"Even though I feel terrible right now, I might be able to feel better."

You say this statement three times, for emphasis. Notice that again, the wording doesn't have to be exact. The three statements can all be the same, or you can vary them. If you are very anxious, for instance if your SUDS is a ten out of ten, you don't even have to say anything; just tap on the karate chop spot.

Now you tap on the points. You want to tap about eight times on each point. However, you don't want to count the number of taps – just guess. If you're counting the taps, you're focused on the process, not on the problem, and this process works on what you're thinking about.

Don't tap too hard – don't give yourself a bruise. And don't tap too gently – you want to let the body know you're there. At the first point, the karate chop point, I use three fingers, as the area is larger.

At all the other points I use two fingers, to make sure I am getting the right spot.

You have an area about the size of a quarter at each point, so you don't have to be right on the point. If you want to make sure you're getting the points right, or if you're just curious, you can get an acupuncture point finder. They are available at acupuncture supply stores – I got a couple of different ones on Amazon. These gadgets are like a Geiger counter for tapping spots, measuring the electrical resistance at various spots on the skin. They beep, and when they locate the right spot, where you want to tap, they beep louder and faster. These devices are a big hit in our tapping classes. I suspect people are relieved to find proof that the points exist, and that we are not just making them up.

This process works on what you are thinking about. So to make sure you're addressing the problem you want to deal with, you will name the problem at each tapping point. You said a longer version at the setup, but for the rest of the tapping points you just use the shorthand words; so, "this stress" or "bill worries."

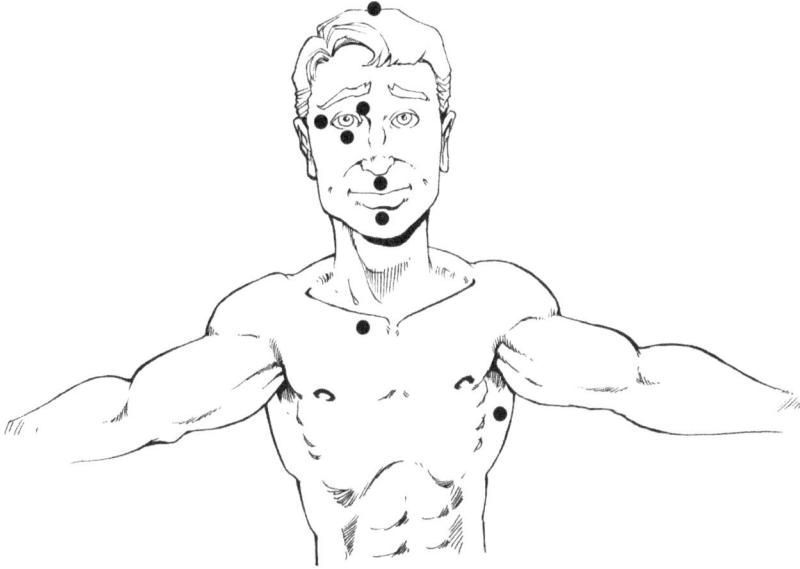

The setup, done on the karate chop point, is first. After that, you can tap the points in any order. To make it easier to remember all the points, I will list them here from the top down.

Top of head

The next thing is to tap on the top of your head. This point is in the middle of your head – halfway between the front and the back of your head and halfway between the left and the right side. It is about where the soft spot would be on an infant's head. If you want, you can tap around a bit so you make sure you get the right spot.

You tap on this point about eight times, more or less, and say your shorthand phrase such as, "this stress."

Eyebrow point

Then you tap on the beginning of your eyebrow. This point is at the inside corner of your eyebrow, where the eyebrow begins. If you feel in that area, you can feel a little dimple in the bone, on the underside of the bony rim over your eye. That's the spot you want to tap while you say your reminder phrase, "this stress." For these points you can tap on the right side, left side, or both sides at the same time. The "sweet spot" is about the size of a quarter, so you don't have to be exact.

Side of eye point

The next spot is on the side of the eye. It is on the outside corner of the eye, at the edge of the bone. Again, you can do the right side or the left side or both at the same time.

Under eye point

Next, you tap under the eye, on the edge of the bone just under your pupil.

Under nose point

The next spot, the under nose point, is in the middle of your upper lip just below your nose. Tap eight times and say your short reminder phrase.

Chin point

The chin point is not really on your chin, but halfway between your lower lip and the point of your chin, where there is an indentation. You tap on that spot while you repeat your reminder phrase.

Collarbone point

The collarbone point is a little tricky for some people. It may help to look at the diagram. There is a notch at the top of your breastbone. Put your finger on that notch. Then move your finger down an inch and to the side an inch, either direction, right or left. You will be right on the collarbone point. For this point it is an advantage that we have such a big area, the size of a quarter, so you don't have to be directly on it.

Underarm point

The underarm point is on either side, four inches under your armpit, about where a woman's bra strap would hit. You can reach across to the other side or tap on the same side. Tap about eight times while repeating the reminder phrase.

Repeat SUDS

Now think about the problem again, and give a SUDS after you've done the tapping. Compare this number to the pre-tapping number.

To review, these are the steps in the basic tapping process:
- Identify the problem
- Give it a SUDS rating from one (least intense) to ten (most intense)
- Tap on the karate chop point while you say what the problem is, and then something like "I'm open to the possibility that it could get better." Repeat the phrase three times, using your own words.
- Name the problem in one or two words while you tap on the following points:
  o Top of head
  o Eyebrow
  o Side of eye
  o Under eye
  o Under nose

- o Chin point
- o Collar bone point
- o Underarm point
- Think about the problem and give it a SUDS again.

Most of the time you will see improvement with just the above points. However, sometimes you will need to use the hand points. Here is the diagram again:

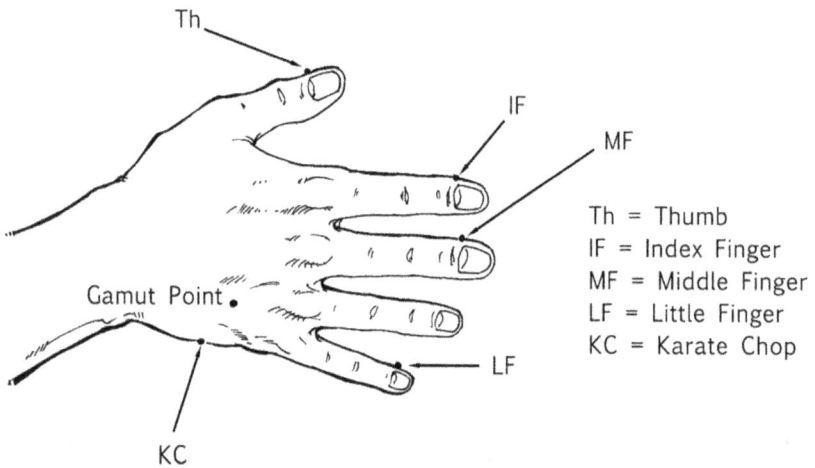

Th = Thumb
IF = Index Finger
MF = Middle Finger
LF = Little Finger
KC = Karate Chop

If you hold your hand with your palm facing your stomach, the tapping points will be on the top of each of these fingers next to the base of the fingernail. Tap on the side of the thumb about eight times while you repeat the short reminder phrase. Then you tap on the index finger, followed by the middle finger. You can skip the ring finger. You tap on the little finger and then tap on the karate chop point while repeating the reminder phrase.

The reason you skip the ring finger is that the ring finger and the karate chop point are on the same meridian, so the ring finger is unnecessary. However, it won't hurt anything if you do tap it. When I am showing someone how to tap, I often tap on all the fingers because it takes less time to tap on the ring finger than it does to explain why I'm omitting it!

You may see a drop in SUDS after the first round, or you may not. Occasionally we get what Gary Craig calls a "one-minute wonder" in which the SUDS goes to zero after the first round and the problem never recurs. That is rare, but it does happen.

If the SUDS is not zero, keep doing several more rounds and check the SUDS after each round. If it doesn't go down, check Chapter 10, "What If It Doesn't Work?"

I used the Ancient Secret with a woman in her fifties who had a problem with hoarding. She had difficulty getting rid of things like old newspapers, in addition to things that once had meaning to her. She had very little room in her house to move around – she was even unable to cook in her kitchen because of all the clutter. We worked together on her fear about throwing things out or giving them away. In a very short time she had cleaned out her house and was preparing to sell it. She planned to move to the place where she really wanted to live. She was able to change her life when her stress about clearing clutter was reduced.

When I do group demonstrations of EFT, I often work with phobias, because the effect is quick and dramatic. At one physicians' meeting I did a demonstration with a psychiatrist who had a fear of snakes. He gave his fear a SUDS of ten. He remembered an incident in his childhood when he watched his father kill a snake by chopping it with a hoe. After we did a few rounds of EFT his SUDS was a zero – he no longer had a fear of snakes.

Being a clerk in a medical office is a stressful job, never more so than at a mental health clinic. Besides checking patients in, notifying the provider, scheduling appointments, and answering the constantly ringing telephone, clerks often have to tell patients what they don't want to hear. Sometimes patients get angry or even violent.

That happened to a clerk in our VA mental health clinic. A patient got angry and decided to charge at the clerk, whom we'll call Darlene. She was behind a window and door, in the clerk's area, with only one exit. The patient tried to open the door to get into the room, and Darlene stood with her shoulder against the door from the inside. It was several minutes before the VA police arrived and escorted the veteran out, to face attempted assault charges.

I happened to come by at that time, and could see that Darlene was extremely upset, shaking, almost unable to talk. We sat down and tapped. We didn't do the setup phrase and I didn't even ask her to say anything; we just kept tapping around the points until she felt calmer, which only took about five minutes.

Chapter 4
Acupuncture Comes to the United States

When President Nixon went to China in 1972, a journalist for the New York Times, James Reston, went along. While he was in China, he had to have surgery to have his appendix removed. After the surgery he had pain, which was treated with acupuncture. When he returned to the United States he wrote about acupuncture and the good results he had with it. You can read his July 26, 1971 New York Times story here: http://www.acupuncture.com/testimonials/restonexp.htm

Reston's story, we would say these days, went viral. Acupuncture became fashionable. A psychologist, Dr. Roger Callahan, began studying the procedure. One day he was seeing a client who had stomach problems that weren't being resolved with psychotherapy. On impulse, he reached over and tapped on the acupuncture meridian that related to the stomach. Instantly, her symptoms improved.

This began Dr. Callahan's Thought Field Therapy. TFT uses tapping on the meridians to relieve a variety of symptoms. For TFT, there is a specific protocol for each symptom; you tap on a list of meridians in a specific order. And so you will usually need to go to a TFT practitioner who knows the algorithm for your specific problem.

I was first introduced to tapping when my colleague, Dr. Audrey Hoo, told me about TFT, which she had learned in graduate school. She told me about Dr. Callahan's book, *Five Minute Phobia Cure*, which I found intriguing, as phobias are notoriously hard to treat. I bought the book and began experimenting with it. And it worked, most of the time. I was puzzled about why more people, more mental health professionals, didn't know about this.

I began trying the protocols on friends, coworkers, family, and anyone who would sit still long enough. One of my coworkers had an addiction to a particular candy bar she would buy every day. We spent five minutes tapping for that candy bar. From that day on, she no longer ate that candy. She just stopped buying it because she just wasn't interested in it anymore.

Craig and EFT

Gary Craig is a Stanford-trained engineer who learned Roger Callahan's TFT technique. From this he developed EFT, Emotional Freedom technique. With Callahan's TFT, there is a different tapping protocol for every problem. But with Gary Craig's newer version, EFT, the tapping technique is the same for any symptom – you tap all the meridians. The process is so quick that it takes little time to hit all the major points. In this way you can be sure you got the relevant energy meridian. So anyone can use the technique without memorizing a long list of protocols for each problem.

This was what I was looking for. People can do EFT on their own. They can get the benefit of acupuncture for free, without needles, even in the middle of the night if they need to. Usually they can find benefit without having to go to an expert. Some nine years later, I find it even more amazing – and often life-changing. I hope it can be life-changing for you.

A few years ago I did some tapping on the telephone with my aunt, Donna Payne, after she had surgery on her knee. EFT helped – her pain improved and the swelling went down right away. For years she didn't use it, but she recently sent me this note:

"Several months ago, I was put on five different heart medicines. As a result, all I wanted to do was sleep and sleep some more. I would get up in the morning after about seven or eight hours of sleep, be up for several hours and then feel the need for a nap. After lunch and several hours in the afternoon, I would feel the need for an afternoon nap, which usually lasted for one to two hours. I was always able to go to bed in the evening and be able to sleep for the night. During the day, it seemed as though any time I sat down, I would go to sleep. I was sleeping my life away!

"After many discouraging months, I presented this information to the doctor and he did decrease the dosage of one of the medications. But the lower dosage did nothing for the sleeping problem. And, I continued to want to nap all the time.

"Finally, I read an article in the publication *Bottom Line* about EFT. I remembered what you had taught me about tapping and decided it was definitely worth a try. So, twice a day, at night before going to bed and in the morning, immediately upon awakening, before doing anything else, I would do the tapping procedure. I found it so important to do this immediately upon getting up. I would move from my bed to the computer chair, get comfortable and do my daily mantra, before anything else. As I tapped each of the spots, I would repeat – 'I am completely and honestly refreshed and energized.' AND, IT WORKED! I am now able to get through the day without napping. It is absolutely a life-saver. In fact, one day, I had a lull in my daily activities and made a decision to take a nap and much to my surprise, when I got in my recliner, I was actually unable to sleep, because my mind was alert and thinking of what was next to be done.

"Now that I am not sleeping the day away, it is amazing what I am able to accomplish and get done during the day. And how much better I feel now that I'm not sleeping most of the day. I definitely attribute this newfound energy to my tapping exercise – especially in the morning."

Chapter 5
If This Is So Great,
Why Have I Never Heard of It?

The women of Vienna were terrified. They would cry and beg the doctor not to assign them to the First Clinic to have their babies, where so many women died after childbirth, but to admit them to the Second Clinic. They were so afraid that many would deliver their own babies in the street and then come to the hospital.

The year was 1847. Dr. Ignaz Semmelweiss, the assistant to the professor of the maternity clinic at the Vienna General Hospital, was puzzled by this problem. The fatality rate in the First Clinic was 10%, while in the Second Clinic it was less than 4%. Even more puzzling, the street deliveries were safer than the First Clinic. Women who delivered in the street had a fatality rate equal to that of the Second Clinic.

In the First Clinic, the babies were delivered by medical students who came directly from doing autopsies. The Second Clinic was staffed by midwives, who didn't do autopsies. Although the germ theory of disease was not yet in favor, Dr. Semmelweiss ordered the medical students to wash their hands with chlorinated lime solution after doing autopsies and before delivering babies. The fatality rate in the First Clinic immediately fell to match the Second Clinic.

What was the reaction of the medical community to this dramatic success? Dr. Semmelweiss was fired from the hospital and forced to move out of Vienna, back to Budapest. He continued to insist that cleanliness was key to medical treatment. Other doctors, and even his wife, believed that he was insane. Eventually he was committed to a mental hospital, where he died two weeks later, after being beaten by guards.

It was only later that Dr. Louis Pasteur proved that indeed infection was the cause of much disease. The Vienna students had bacteria from the autopsied patients on their hands and transferred the infection to the women, who then died of puerperal fever.

Why was Dr. Semmelweiss so dramatically unsuccessful in convincing the profession to simply wash their hands? Frantz Fanon explains: "Sometimes people hold a core belief that is very strong. When they are presented with evidence that works against that belief, the new evidence cannot be accepted. It would create a feeling that is extremely uncomfortable, called cognitive dissonance. And because it is so important to protect the core belief, they will rationalize, ignore and even deny anything that doesn't fit in with the core belief."

The Vienna doctors didn't believe it was possible that tiny creatures were causing the puerperal fever, so they ignored the clear evidence that they were, to the detriment of their patients.

We all have our understanding of the world and how it operates, what is true and what is not. And our assumptions work for us, more or less, most of the time. But when we are presented with something that goes against our worldview, we may dismiss it as nonsense. Thomas Kuhn famously explained this principle in effect in science. When the scientific community holds a particular belief, no amount of evidence is enough to get most of them to change those beliefs. In *The Structure of Scientific Revolutions*, he introduced the term "paradigm" to describe the overall concepts, the underlying framework of beliefs that we use. When something new comes along that challenges our previous views, we don't just adopt the new belief. We have to have a "paradigm shift," to change our whole notion of what is possible, in order to make room for the new information. This is difficult, and Kuhn said that generally science has to wait until the old generation dies off before the new paradigm will take hold.

Olga probably still has not heard of EFT. Why did the clinic supervisor ban me from using it? She said at the time that another patient complained. None of us believed that excuse. Certainly patients complain all the time about a whole lot of things. But if that was how we operated, then a patient who didn't like Prozac could complain about our using it. We would then forbid everyone to use Prozac despite the fact that many people were getting benefit from it.

No, the truth is that the supervisor was a fan of another therapy technique. Ironically, Olga's symptoms were too severe at the time for her to benefit from the supervisor's favorite therapy process.

The question of acceptance by the medical community is complicated. A few years ago, I went to work at a large clinic in a veteran's hospital. The staff were experienced and dedicated, and they were accustomed to using several different treatment methods. I began using EFT with veterans with some success, despite the fact that psychiatrists are only supposed to prescribe medications. Eventually word got out, and other staff members would refer patients to me for EFT. It was only after a year or so that I discovered that many of the staff had actually taken the training for EFT but just didn't use it.

Medicine will need a paradigm shift in order to accept these processes. Fortunately, you don't have to wait for them to catch up. You can use it now.

The Toaster

When acupuncture caught on and became popular, I suspect that part of the appeal was that it went against the established version of the truth. We believed then that Western medicine was the most advanced and most effective form of treatment, and that it was the only game in town – or at least the best game. But if acupuncture could work, maybe we were missing something. Around this time was the beginning of Western fascination with Eastern philosophy, medicine, even theories of what constitutes our body and minds. I believe people started to see that we are not just the toaster.

Let's say you have a toaster. You want the toaster to work well so that it will toast your bread the way you like it. If the toaster is to work, it needs all the right parts: the metal, wiring, the heater element, the spring that pops it up and the other fancy things that you may have paid extra for but don't really need.

But you also need the electricity. It has to be plugged in to an outlet, the outlet has to have electricity running through it, there must be enough current, and the electricity has to go to the right places. Otherwise the toaster won't work, or it won't work correctly.

I believe this is why acupuncture had such an impact in the West. Western medicine focuses on the parts of the toaster, makes sure that they are all in working order, that they're in the right place and in good

25

condition. We pay much less attention to the power that flows through the toaster.

We do acknowledge that there is electricity in the body, and that it is important. When you do an EKG, for instance, it measures the electrical activity in your heart; the same with an EEG or EMG which measures electrical activity in your brain or muscles. But for the most part, Western medicine is toaster medicine. We tend to deny the importance of the electricity, saying that if it can't be seen or measured, it doesn't exist. Or if elaborate, expensive studies have not been done to prove something, it doesn't work. Drug companies claim that it takes a billion dollars to do all the work to get a new medication approved – to go through all the studies that are required. Anything, such as acupuncture, which can't possibly come up with a billion dollars for such a study, is denigrated as "pseudoscience." That is interpreted as "it doesn't work" – but it really means "nobody has really investigated it." That is a big difference.

In fact, both the toaster and the electricity are important. Similarly, if you want your computer to work, you need both the hardware and the software.

And so we have the problem of toaster medicine. If we are only the toaster, talking about the electricity makes no sense. Treatment that addresses the electricity is a sham, a fraud.

Dr. Callahan described what he called the Apex problem, where people would see their symptoms improve dramatically after doing TFT, and then deny that the TFT was the cause of the improvement. Sometimes they would even deny that they ever had the problem at all. The reasoning seemed to be, "Since I don't have this problem now, I never had it." I have seen this phenomenon also. People would get rapid, obvious improvement in stress, and then would deny that the tapping worked.

Medicine believes that our industry is driven by evidence, but that is only partly true. It is also driven by belief systems, and our current paradigm is that people are the toaster – they are only their bodies. Even psychiatry has gone toaster. We used to call our profession mental health, and would focus on the mind. Now we have behavioral health, addressing only behaviors, not the mind and certainly not the person. We treat brain chemistry.

There is plenty of evidence for EFT. You can look online for the research. TFT has been officially accepted as having evidence of its efficacy, and the growing EFT research will soon meet that standard. But what proof do you need to try it? It's just a matter of tapping on specific spots for a few minutes. If it doesn't work, what have you lost?

Chapter 6
More About EFT

The EFT process can be as complicated as you want to make it, but at its heart it is very simple. The basic version takes five minutes to learn, and it is often all you need to help your stress. Like anything else, there are tricks and modifications, but if the simple version works, you didn't need anything more elaborate or complicated. Whether I am using the tapping for myself or someone else, I do the short version first. If it works, that is all that is needed. If the short version doesn't work, I add other strategies.

The first response I often get from people is "That's weird." I hear it so often that I say it myself to them first: "I know, it's weird, right?" I say this as they have a puzzled look on their face, because their problem has changed – and maybe disappeared.

Many people feel a tingling, or a feeling of warmth or rushing. Western medicine has no explanation for this, although it is a repeatable phenomenon ("scientific," if you will.) The explanation given by acupuncturists is that when you were feeling more stressed, the flow of energy was blocked. The tapping unblocks the energy meridian and you now feel the energy flow. You may find yourself yawning or sighing – that's a good sign. It means the energy meridian is aligning.

You may find that one point seems to work better for you than the others. There are multiple energy meridians, or pipelines, and they are not likely all out of balance. There may be only one meridian that is out of balance at that time, for that symptom, and you may only need to tap that one point. If you feel a twinge or other sensation at one of the points, or one has more effect than others, this may indicate that further tapping on that point would be helpful.

You may be looking up other teachers of the tapping technique and online videos – I hope you are. And you may notice that they do the setup differently. As Gary Craig teaches it, the setup phrase is, "Even though I have (this problem), I deeply and completely love and accept myself." You can certainly use this phrase in your tapping if you choose. The reason I don't teach it is that so many people have a problem with that statement – they don't love themselves, or don't believe they do, and just saying something they don't believe to be true can interfere with the process.

If I am working individually with someone, I may use this "deeply and completely" phrase. Then if he or she has a negative reaction to the statement, we can deal with that. Otherwise I prefer to use the "open to the possibility" phrase I described above.

Some symptoms come down quickly – for example, SUDS ratings after each round can be nine, then six, then two, then zero. Other symptoms come down very slowly – one-half point to one point per round, and no decrease at all on some rounds. I can't tell you why that is so, but I can tell you that they do.

My colleague Rachel Bensinger and I were teaching a group of veterans this process to help them deal with post-traumatic stress disorder. One of the veterans reported that she had an extreme fear of spiders and would panic whenever she saw one. We tapped on "this fear of spiders" and immediately her fear vanished. She was able to handle a plastic spider without any feeling at all, saying, "That's interesting."

This is an example of what Gary Craig calls a "one-minute wonder," when we tap on the issue for one or two rounds and the problem disappears and never returns. While this is not the most common experience, it happens frequently. It is not a surprise to EFT therapists, although it is usually startling to the person doing the tapping, who may find it strange to have that familiar feeling suddenly disappear.

Chapter 7
I'm Stressed Now

I certainly hope you never have an attempted assault the way Darlene did, but if you do, EFT is something you can use to help reduce the panic. You will more likely have the usual stresses of daily modern life. You can use EFT any time when you get anxious, worried, or fearful. You can use it when other people are being annoying or ridiculous. It won't change them, but it will make your day better. You can use it in the middle of the night when you can't sleep or had a fearful dream. You can use it when you are worried about your child.

You can use EFT after something happens that makes you feel upset. But you can also use it in advance, to prevent worry and fear. So you can use it before you have to speak in front of a group or have to give your boss bad news.

What is your usual stress reliever? Is it healthy? Is it calling a friend or meditating or going for a run? Or is it something more unhealthy? Stress relievers are very individual. You know if yours is healthy or not. A glass of wine is not the same as a bottle of wine. There's playing a video game, and there's playing a video game all day. Alcohol, binge shopping, driving too fast: you can use EFT as a substitute for those more unhealthy habits.

Try a round or two of EFT if you're feeling as if you are at the end of your rope. Are you feeling overwhelmed, lost, abandoned, guilty, fearful, in pain, can't get past the hurt, seeing no way out of a bad situation, nothing is going right? I have seen people get relief from all of these feelings, some more than others.

But also try it when you're at the *middle* of your rope – when you have everyday worries, when you can't sleep and the day keeps playing out in your mind, when you are overwhelmed and too busy, when your children need more than you can give them, when you can't be yourself and you don't know how to fix what is wrong. If you do this, you may prevent ordinary problems from becoming bigger problems. But in addition, you may start to feel more in charge of your life.

I am not a big fan of affirmations. I believe they don't work for most people because we don't really believe what we are saying. Most of us are likely to find them ineffective, most of the time. One of the things I like about EFT is that we don't have to believe anything. We can complain out loud and tap while we're doing it and often find relief from the symptoms. So when you are feeling "normal" stress, try tapping and see what it can do for you. I challenge you to try it for ten minutes every day for ten days, and let me know whether you see any results.

One of the first comments I get when I am demonstrating EFT is that it looks strange, and people don't want anyone else to see them doing it. If you don't want someone to see you tapping, you can do what we call "Touch and Breathe." In this technique you touch the first tapping spot, at the beginning of the eyebrow. You hold your finger there while you take a normal breathing cycle – breathe in normally, then breathe out normally. Don't take a deep breath; breathe as you always do. Then move on to the next point, the outside corner of the eye. Put your finger on the tapping spot and hold it there while you breathe normally, in and out. Repeat this for each of the tapping spots. There is no hurry; you can leave your finger on the point for as long as you want.

Another option is to imagine yourself tapping. You can do this when you are lying in bed, half asleep, and don't want to move your arm. For this process you imagine yourself tapping the spots, repeating the reminder phrase silently to yourself. This can also be useful when you are in a public situation. Let's say you are at work when your boss is demanding something unreasonable – you can imagine you are tapping and nobody is any the wiser.

In this chapter, we talked about relieving stress in the current moment, about feeling better now. Tapping can often help you feel better right away. It often helps day to day, moment to moment. However, for chronic stress, you may have better results with a different approach.

Chapter 8
I'm Always Stressed

EFT can help when you are stressed in the moment, when something unexpected arises, or for one-time problems. You can tap to deal with stresses in the present. But you can also use it for ongoing, chronic stress; more recurrent issues, such as chronic anxiety, phobias, feeling stressed every time you interact with your boss, or frustration when you have to deal with your annoying neighbor.

You may have stress that keeps coming up. Often, past issues affect the now. EFT can often help resolve old events that have become a long-standing problem. Events from our past can take our time and energy; and interfere with our life, our happiness, and our peace and contentment. Old problems can interfere with who we are and how we live our lives.

Even if we believe our reaction is "normal," it is still a problem. Whatever happens on the outside affects the inside. Many of us are used to just putting up with such problems. We believe it is best to just power through it, but it takes a toll on our energy and even our happiness. If there is a tool you can use to deal with the stress, you may decide it is better to stop and address it.

You may feel powerless to deal with stress – many people do. Those who become accustomed to a stressed life may believe that there is no other option. My suggestion is that you try tapping, both for inside and outside stressors. You have nothing to lose except a few minutes, and it costs nothing. You may be surprised at the results. If you learn that there is something you can do, you will feel more in control, less powerless.

When you have chronic stress, you may need to be more focused and more persistent. Persistence makes this technique more effective. If you try it for just a few minutes every day, the effect can be stronger.

Again, it works best to tap for a specific incident, so be as specific as you can. If you say "I'm always stressed" you may not find much improvement. If you tap on, "Each time I hear my neighbor's voice I get angry," you may have somewhat better success. But you are most likely to see improvement if you say something like, "I am angry at my neighbor because of the time I saw him kick my dog." The more specific you can be, the more likely you will see results.

For another example, if you say, "My boss drives me crazy," you may or may not have good results. if you say "I get a sick feeling every morning when I have to go to work" you may have a better result. If you say, "I am so angry at my boss because she moved my office." you may have even more improvement.

If you say "I am so afraid to drive on the freeway," you may not see much improvement. If you say "that time I got a flat tire on the freeway," you may have better results.

To make this clearer:
Good: "I'm always stressed."
Better: "Each time I hear my neighbor's voice I get angry."
Best: "That time my neighbor kicked my dog."

For another example,
Good: "My boss drives me crazy."
Better: "I get a sick feeling every morning when I have to go to work."
Best: "When my boss moved my office."

Good: "Driving is stressful."
Better: "I am afraid to drive on the freeway."
Best: "That time I got a flat tire on the freeway."

In general, the earlier in your life the incident took place that you are tapping on, the more effect it is likely to have on your current and future stress. Often we are tapping on what seems to be a clear incident, such as getting a flat tire on the freeway, and not seeing much improvement. When this happens, I will ask, "Is there something earlier in your life that this reminds you of?" And maybe the person will remember wrecking a bicycle and getting unfairly scolded for it. So if we tap for the earlier bicycle incident, the freeway fear may be reduced.

I have to mention a couple of childhood events that are strikingly common and influential on adult lives. One is something like, "the time the third-grade teacher called me stupid." I am amazed at how often I hear a story like this and how it affects so many people. The other one is particularly in common in men. This is, "that time the coach said I couldn't do anything right." If one of these is a memory for you, you might want to do some tapping for it. This could have an effect on your stress. If you are a coach or a teacher, or if you know a coach or a teacher, please pass on the information that their statements can have a powerful effect on children, for good or for bad. What they say can have an effect, years or even decades later.

We don't change history. We can't change the teachers and coaches in the past who said hurtful things. But we can change how you react to it and how it affects your stress today. You can't change clueless bosses and careless neighbors, but you can change whether you let them get to you. After all, you know people who don't let things bother them. Maybe you can be one of them.

If you are tapping on a general problem and do not remember a specific incident, that's okay. Start with the general, "I always get anxious when I think about going to work," and give the anxiety level a SUDS. Tap on it, and sometimes a specific event will come to mind.

You may be able to identify a trigger that makes your stress worse. This can be a time of day, a physical location, or an event. So for instance, nighttime can be a difficult time for some – nighttime can be a trigger for overeating or drinking. Perhaps there is an event earlier in life that happened at night that is triggering this stress.

A trigger can be a location. So, for instance, driving over a bridge can bring on fear or panic. Or a trigger can be an event such as someone criticizing you or making a racist statement. If there is such an event for you, you can tap on this ongoing problem. If you can tie it to something that happened when you were younger, you may have better results.

If you have an incident in your past that is traumatic, EFT can help. However, if you have a Big-T Trauma, I do not recommend that you try to deal with it yourself. I suggest you work with a therapist, for several reasons. We all have things in our past that we minimize, and put away in the closet, then shut the door and try to live as if it didn't happen. When you do the tapping, that closet door may open and the event may come out, demanding to be dealt with. If it is a small-t trauma, we have an opportunity to clean out the closet and make the problem not be a problem anymore. But if it is a Big-T Trauma, it can be overpowering, more than we can handle by ourselves. That is why I recommend that you work with a therapist.

Another reason for a therapist, for any size issue, is that they can be more objective. When we are focusing on the problem, we may have a limited perspective. A therapist can usually see the broader picture, suggest things that we may not be aware of, or even give feedback on our body language and way of speaking that can give clues to solutions to the problem.

The Writing on our Walls

Stress can come from early life events, or it can come from your assumptions and approach to life. We are all taught things in childhood from our parents, teachers and coaches, and others. Gary Craig calls this "the writing on our walls." So, "Our family doesn't do that." Or "The world isn't safe." A common wall message is "I am unworthy." Another is "Money is evil/bad/dirty/unspiritual."

Most of the things we learned are helpful to keep us safe or navigate this crazy world. So we learn to "look before you cross the road" or "brush your teeth twice a day," and this benefits us. The trick is to separate those writings from the ones that are getting in the way.

I often hear from people that, "I was an adult before I realized that not everyone thinks that way." And one of the tasks of adulthood is to review what we learned, and choose which messages to keep and which to discard. But shedding old messages can be a challenge, and this is another way that EFT can be helpful. If, for instance, unworthiness is a gremlin for you, you can tap on the feeling in the moment and it may diminish. You are likely to have better results if you can identify a time when you were told or reminded about your unworthiness. The earlier in your life this event happened, the more likely it is that tapping will reduce its effect on you today and in the future.

Phobias

Phobias often respond well to EFT. I was introduced to tapping when my coworker told me about Roger Callahan's book, *Five Minute Phobia Cure*. This book demonstrates TFT, and I now use EFT instead, but the principles, and the reason it works, are the same.

Unless you have a Big-T Trauma associated with a phobia, you can address your phobia by yourself. If the SUDS goes down, you may want to test it with a plastic spider or snake. If it doesn't work, you are probably dealing with different aspects, a topic I will address in Chapter 10, "What if it Doesn't Work?"

Insomnia

Insomnia can have multiple causes. If you're drinking caffeine late in the day, EFT probably won't help. But if anxiety or worry is keeping you awake, give it a try. Before you go to bed you can tap for whatever the experience is: "I feel stressed," or "I always toss and turn," or "I am worried about my brother's surgery tomorrow."

At night I like to imagine myself tapping, rather than raising my arm and doing physical tapping, but do what works for you. You can tap for "this leg pain" or "these racing thoughts." Before you go to sleep you can tap through the points, saying "I choose to sleep well tonight. I choose to have restful, peaceful sleep throughout the night."

You don't always have to use tapping on something that you don't want. Tapping can also be used to achieve something that you *do* want. So you can tap for "this trouble falling asleep" but you can also tap for "falling asleep quickly and sleeping soundly." You can tap for "getting that great job." Tapping is good for sports performance, "beating my personal best time tomorrow." Margaret Lynch has some great videos online for "tapping for miracles" and even "tapping for $50,000."

Dr. Pat Carrington has developed a very effective method she calls the Choices Method. For this process, you tap for a round on the problem, and then tap for a round on what you prefer. So you would tap on "I get stressed when I drive on the freeway." Then you tap for "I choose to be calm when I drive." Then you do a round alternating the two. So:

One round of "I get stressed when I drive on the freeway."
One round of "I choose to be calm when I drive."

Then:
Eyebrow: "Stress on the freeway"
Side of eye: "I choose to be calm when I drive."
Under eye: "Stress on the freeway"
Under nose: "I choose to be calm when I drive."
Chin: "Stress on the freeway"
Collarbone: "I choose to be calm when I drive."
Under arm: "Stress on the freeway"
Top of head: "I choose to be calm when I drive."

If you have worries about an upcoming job interview, you could tap on "I am so stressed out about this interview." Then you would tap on "I choose to be relaxed during the interview." The last round would alternate the two statements.

Affirmations, as I have mentioned, are often ineffective because we don't believe what we are saying – for example, "I am now calm and relaxed." But in the Choices Method, we are making a statement that we do believe – we do choose to be relaxed, even when we aren't. It is important that you are saying something that you believe. So if it doesn't feel right to say, "I choose to be relaxed," you can use your own words. So, you could say:

"I could be relaxed."
"It is possible that I could relax."
"I'm open to the possibility that I could relax."
"Maybe I could give up some of this stress."
"Maybe this could happen."
"I would rather feel calm."

Or whatever feels comfortable to you. All of these would be fine.

Let's say you are stressed about bills. You could tap for one round on, "these bills." Or "I am stressed about these bills." Then you can tap on "I could be relaxed about these bills." Or "I choose to give up some of this stress about bills." Then the last round would alternate the two statements.

Persistence

EFT can be dramatically helpful for reducing stress. Sometimes we see a one-minute wonder, and that particular issue is never a problem for you again. But most of the time it helps to be persistent. So if you tap for five or ten minutes a day, twice a day if possible, you may see a gradual improvement in your stress level.

Chapter 9

What Do I Say?

A frequent concern that people have is that they are not saying the right thing. In fact, the words you use are not as important as what you're thinking and feeling. Dr. Callahan called his treatment method "Thought Field Therapy" because it works on what you're thinking. So your thoughts are the key – and your words keep you focused on the problem, rather than being distracted by other thoughts. However, many people worry about saying the right thing.

At the end of this chapter, I will provide some suggestions for scripts to follow when you are tapping for stress. Some therapists and EFT practitioners are not in favor of scripts for tapping. They say they are not effective, and Gary Craig warns against them. I understand the concern. Since tapping scripts are not your own words but someone else's, they may not work as well as using your own words. But people who are new to tapping want to know what to say, and many worry about getting the words just right. There is a big demand for such scripts because people often feel uncertain about this technique, which is a completely new approach to stress. They may feel awkward and uncertain about the words to use.

The easiest and simplest thing to do is to just describe what you're feeling. So "I feel awful" is a perfectly good thing to say, or "this terrible feeling." You can say "this stress" or you can say "I am so fed up right now." You can swear. Really, it's okay.

For the setup phrase, which is used at the beginning when tapping on the karate chop point, some go into a long description. I tend to make it a bit more brief, just a couple of sentences. Either is fine.

A longer version would be: "Even though my mother put me in the closet and told me I had to stay there all day and I was really terrified and I couldn't breathe and I just kept crying and I still can't go into an elevator, I'm open to the possibility that I could have less fear." Some EFT practitioners use a very long setup, describing the problem in detail, various associated thoughts, feelings, and descriptions, and the desired outcome.

I usually use a shorter setup, such as: "Even though my mother put me in the closet, I could give up some of this fear."

Another longer setup might be: "Even though Miss Flanagan made fun of me in front of the fourth grade class and now I hate getting up in front of a group to talk, I need to make a presentation to the board next week, and maybe I can do it calmly."

A shorter setup might be: "Even though Miss Flanagan made fun of me, I am open to the possibility that I can let go of this fear of speaking."

Then for the tapping round, use a couple of words that say what the problem is or what the feeling is. So, "this fear" or "that talk to the group" or "driving over the bridge."

If you're unsure of what to say, just pretend you're talking to a friend and telling her what the problem is. Use your own words. If you have difficulty coming up with words, just say "this feeling" or "this bad feeling" or "I feel terrible."

You can say the same reminder phrase at each tapping point, "this stress, this stress, this stress." However, I find that my mind often wanders. So I find it holds my attention better if I change the words around a little bit, "this stress, I'm feeling stressed, tired of feeling stressed, ready to let it all go," etc.

You may want to exaggerate what you're saying; just exaggerating your feelings can give you a different perspective on the problem. And you can use humor. So, you can tap on "I ate too much, I feel so bloated and uncomfortable, I'm sure I gained twenty pounds today. I'm not going to eat another thing for a week." When you use humor or exaggeration you don't feel as stuck – you understand that you are bigger than the problem. This can help give you hope that there will be a solution.

Talk and Tap

A simple thing to do is just to tap through the points while you tell the story of what happened and how that is affecting you now. This is called "talk and tap." So you will tap through the points while you tell what went on that you find upsetting. You might say, "I was walking my dog and going by the neighbor's house and he came out and started yelling at me. He got so mad and then he kicked my dog. I'm just so upset. I can't believe somebody would do that." So while you tell that story you just tap through the points.

When you're focused on the story and not the points, you may not hit all the tapping points – you may skip one or two. Don't worry about it. This is a very forgiving process.

Some people find it easy to describe their feelings; others don't. Some are better than others at being sensitive to their feelings and being able to put their feelings into words. It is perfectly fine to say "I feel awful" or "this terrible feeling."

Different people experience the world and themselves differently. Some people perceive visually. Others are auditory – their best source of information is what they hear. Some are kinesthetic and experience by feeling. How do you experience your stress? Do you see it as a color, do you hear it, or do you feel in your body?

If you *see* your stress, you may see an animal or even a blob. Perhaps you see "this big fiery monster coming toward me" or "the squirrel chewing up money." It is common for people to see their stress as a color. I have had patients describe to me that the problem looks fiery red, or sometimes a dull brown. So you would tap for "this bright-red lump," or "this dull, heavy, brown stress."

Or do you feel your stress in your body? It is common to feel stress in the stomach or between the shoulder blades. Do you feel a knot in your shoulder, a heaviness in your stomach, a headache, or nausea? You can tap for "this heaviness on my shoulders" or "this bowling ball in my stomach."

Constricted Breathing

When we are stressed, our breathing becomes shallow. An effective way to tap for stress is called the constricted breathing technique. For this technique, you take a deep breath and rate the breath from one to ten, where ten is the deepest breath possible and one is the shallowest. You don't need to do the karate chop setup; just tap around the points saying "this constricted breathing, this shallow breathing, this breathing." Then take another deep breath, and rate this on the SUDS scale. Even though this doesn't consciously focus on stress, it often helps you feel calmer.

Negative Thoughts

Some people aren't comfortable with tapping because it asks them to focus on the problem, to repeat the problem over and over while they tap. Many other stress-reduction techniques teach that negative thoughts produce more negative thoughts and insist that you not think negatively.

However, EFT is different. With tapping, we can reduce the impact of negative thoughts – and often abolish them entirely. So you need to bring them up, and have them in your awareness, in order to reduce them. I see it like cleaning out a closet – you have to open the closet door first if you want to clean it out.

Tapping Scripts

You can find many tapping scripts available online and for sale. One or several of them may work for you. They may be helpful, but you are likely to do much better creating your own words. Words are very individual. I find when working with someone, I do better using their own words rather than my interpretation of them. No two of us speak alike, and words have meaning to us.

Here's a suggested script for tapping. Use your own words.

"Even though I'm feeling stressed – and I feel hopeless and frustrated, that nothing is ever going to change – maybe I could feel a little better."

"Even though I'm stressed today, it could get better."

"Even though I'm really, really stressed and panicking, I'm open to the possibility that this feeling could get better."

Tapping on the points

"The stress, this stress, I'm feeling stressed, I feel awful, I feel so stressed, this stress."

Chapter 10
What if it Doesn't Work?

Sometimes the results of tapping are delayed. Improvements may come minutes or even hours later. You may see gradual improvement over the course of a day or so. However, if you do not see improvement, there are some things you can try.

Drink water

Many of us are chronically dehydrated, especially when we drink caffeinated beverages throughout the day. But dehydration can interfere with healing, whether by tapping or other energy methods. Better hydration can have a positive health effect. If you are not having the effects that you want from tapping, try drinking more water.

Be more specific

The most common reason EFT doesn't work is that you are not being specific enough. If you're using a general statement such as "I always feel stressed," or "I'm so sad," you may not be getting results. You may want to try a more specific statement, or focus on one specific incident.

A statement like "He makes me so mad" is so general that it probably won't work. Instead, you might try something more specific: "I get upset when someone says something negative about my daughter." Or, "that time he refused to pay for the damage he did."

Earlier event

In general, the earlier in life an event took place, the more effect on your life it has. The younger you were when something happened to you, the more power it can have over you now. If you are not having good luck with tapping, see if you can come up with an earlier life event. When you think of something that is stressful, ask yourself, "What does this remind me of?" "When did something like this happen before?"

So, if you are not seeing improvement when you tap on "I panic when I have to get on an elevator," try an earlier event such as "when I locked myself in the closet when I was six."

Change the setup phrase

I use the setup phrase, "Even though I have this (state the problem), I am open to the possibility that this could get better." I vary the words a bit, but I use statements that are similar. If you are not seeing results, you can try Gary Craig's original setup phrase. He uses "Even though I have (this problem), I deeply and completely love and accept myself anyway."

I usually don't use Gary's statement, at least at first, because so many people say that they really don't love and/or accept themselves. I consider this an affirmation, and affirmations don't work if you don't believe them. However, you can try it and see whether it works better for you. It is a bit of a stronger statement than the one I use. It also forces you to pay attention to your own positive attributes and strengths.

Emphasis

Another thing you can try is to give more emphasis to the words you are using. You can even yell. And as I mentioned in Chapter 9, if you can exaggerate your statements, they have more power. So, if "I am stressed today" is not working, try something like, "I feel awful, and I'm sick of feeling like this, and I'll never feel good again."

Color, sound, feeling

Do you see your stress as a color? Tap for that color. Do you hear it as a sound? Tap on that. Do you feel your stress in your body? Where do you feel it and what does it feel like? Tap for that feeling. So you can tap on:

"This bright red, angry thing in my life."

"This knot in my stomach."

"I keep hearing my mother's voice saying I'll never amount to anything."

Constricted breathing

If you are not getting good results with the basic recipe, you can try the constricted breathing technique I described in Chapter 9. Again, take a deep breath and rate it from one to ten, where ten is the deepest breath possible and one is the shallowest. Then tap around the points, saying, "This constricted breathing, this shallow breathing, this breathing" or similar words. Then take another deep breath and rate this on the SUDS scale.

Tail enders

When you use an affirmation such as "I am happy, wealthy and slender," if you are saying something you don't believe is true, you may have a tail ender. A tail ender is something your mind adds on when you don't believe what you are saying.

So you might say, "I am happy at my job," but your mind adds, "That will never happen." You say, "I feel great," but you think, "Oh no, I don't." A tail ender could be, "That's just not true," or "I can never do that."

When you have a tail ender, you can either change the tapping statement or tap on the tail ender. So perhaps you are tapping on "I am calm today while driving on the freeway," but you are thinking, "No, I'm not." One solution would be to change the tapping statement to "I am stressed when I drive on the freeway." That would be saying something you believe to be true.

Instead of saying "I love my job" when you don't, you could tap on "I dread going to my job." Instead of "I am calm as I give the talk to the board," you could tap on "I get shaky when I have to speak in front of people."

EFT works better when you are tapping on what you actually feel or believe. It helps to focus on your actual feeling. Nick Ortner calls this "truth tapping."

Instead of changing the problem statement, you could tap on the tail ender itself. So you would tap on:

"That will never happen. "

"That is not possible."

"I don't deserve it."

Remember to give it a SUDS before and after you tap. That way, if you see a small decrease, you will still see that something is changing.

A few years ago, Rachel Bensinger and I were doing a group, teaching veterans tapping for PTSD. One of the veterans had good luck with tapping for stress in the class, and he decided to try it outside the group. He had to go into a crowded restaurant, where he felt very anxious. He tapped, saying "I am calm and relaxed. There is nothing to fear." But he had a tail-ender that said, "No I'm not," and the tapping didn't work for him – his anxiety did not improve. In this situation he could have changed the statement to "I'm really stressed," and that would probably have reduced his panic.

Aspects

If you have a traumatic event such as a car wreck, the memory of the wreck may bring up anxiety. Or you may have triggers such as seeing a car of that same model, passing by the site of the wreck, or hearing about someone else's car wreck.

When we tap for an old event, we may need to separate out different aspects of that incident. So the memory includes the sights – what you saw; the smell you remember; how you felt at the time; what someone said just before the wreck, etc. When we use tapping, we may have to separate out these different aspects. If tapping on "the car wreck" isn't helping, we may need to separate out the parts. This may be easier to do with a therapist rather than by yourself.

In another example, a snake phobia may resolve with a couple of rounds of tapping. But if it doesn't, we may need to separate out the look of the snake, how it moves, the sound it makes, and tap on each aspect of the snake or of your fear of the snake.

When you have a previous event that is affecting you today, you may need to separate each of your feelings as a different aspect. So you will make a list of the feelings – anger, fear, sadness, feeling unsafe, resentment, etc., and give each of them a SUDS. Then tap on each aspect separately. Often if one or two decrease in intensity, they will all become less severe.

Chapter 11
What Is the Downside?

Big-T Trauma

Remember Barbara, who remembered a traumatic event whose memory kept her from having surgery? As Joan and I were tapping with Barbara, she got in touch with the panic and the powerlessness that resulted from the event. She started to experience the feelings she felt during the assault. Joan and I are experienced therapists, and we were able to help her work through the panic. We are professionals and we know how to deal with it. But if Barbara had been alone when the feelings arose, it would have been overwhelming for her. This is why I recommend you work with a therapist for a Big-T Trauma. This is not something you want to do on your own.

This is one of the side effects of EFT. Hidden memories may surface, memories that you repressed. Old issues come up when we are doing the tapping. Trauma comes to your awareness, perhaps negative feelings that you weren't even aware of. This is the way the mind protects us. If something is too intense to deal with, it gets tucked away in a closet in the mind/body. Although you may or may not consciously remember the event, it can still be affecting your physical and/or mental health. These traumatic events are actually contributing to stress. This can be an obstacle to healing. You may never have significant improvement in your stress until these memories are dealt with.

Tapping may open the door to where these memories are locked away, whether that is your intention or not. Some see this as a negative side effect, as they would prefer to have the memories stay hidden. However, as therapists we consider it positive, as it is often essential for healing. We acknowledge that it can be uncomfortable, but it is progress. After all, if you want to clean out a closet, you first have to open the door. And yes, you may find a dirtball or two in the closet.

The first session with Barbara was different from the second. In the first session we demonstrated the EFT technique and just dealt with the everyday anxiety of dealing with teenagers and the various stresses of modern life. She then used it at home regularly and was able to change her whole style of dealing with life, to the point that her family remarked on it. They were surprised that she didn't get upset with minor things anymore, and now allowed her teenagers to solve their own problems.

The first session shows the difference between Big-T Trauma and little-t trauma. When the issue is parenting teenagers, EFT is a good thing to try on your own. It helped Barbara – she could have done the first session on her own. The second session was about Big-T Trauma, the assault, and it is preferable to deal with such issues with a therapist.

As in our session with Barbara, EFT will often open the closet door and bring back a memory of a difficult event. Again, we don't change history with this technique; the event still happened. What tapping can often do is to reduce the hold it has on us – the event loses power. So people will be able to say, "Yes, that happened, but it's over now and in the past." Many will find that their anger, fear, resentment and sadness can decrease all the way to zero.

However, if you have a situation where you need to testify in court about that event, your calmness could be used against you. If you no longer have panic and fear, you seem to not be distressed by the event. This can appear as an indication that it never happened, or that you are trying to make it seem worse than it was. You may not be seen as a believable witness.

This is the other downside of EFT. I said earlier that there are almost no side effects from EFT, and that is true. There are, however, two potential risks. The first is that you will open that closet door and the old trauma will come to your attention. The second risk is that if you are no longer suffering emotional consequences of a traumatic incident, you may not convince a courtroom that you have suffered an injury.

Finally, if you are feeling suicidal or out of control during this process for any reason, please get help. If it is an emergency, call 9-1-1. Otherwise, please consult your health care providers. Help is always available.

Joni's Story

I started tapping about one year ago. I had recently sold my home and moved into an apartment. I was having bad anxiety problems, crying a lot, was in severe debt, not working out and very overweight. I was miserable in my job, often driving home crying. I was also having a ton of anxiety about my dogs, being cooped up in the apartment all day. Having to take care of them caused me anxiety.

I spent many weekends totally alone, not seeing anyone but the people at the store where I would go to food shop. By Sunday I was a mess, feeling sorry for myself, so lonely and sad. I was in therapy and sobbed every single session.

All I could think about was how much I lost when my husband died. Everyone else had family but me. All my friends were still in their homes but me.

I was facing loans for the kids. I was having anxiety about my rent going up. I was worried I was going to be on the street with nowhere I could afford to live.

I started tapping off and on and took a weight-loss webinar with Jessica Ortner. I was fairly diligent about doing the classes and doing the meditations in the morning pretty religiously, and I began working out on a somewhat regular basis.

I started to do a number of online tapping webinars that came my way, and I got in touch with my issues around not feeling entitled to have good things happen to me. I tapped on abundance with Carol Look and I did some abundance meditating with Christie Shelton.

My therapist pushed me to call my financial planner and meet with her. She and I decided to pay off everything I owed, to use my retirement funds with no penalty. I paid everything off! It felt good, and scary, at the same time. I would now have to live within what I earned for the first time.

I tapped on all of this, made lunches to stop spending money on lunch every day, and bought nothing that I did not absolutely need. I was able to restrain myself in ways that I have never been able to do before. At the same time, I was starting to work out, doing Zumba at the gym twice a week with a friend. And I was losing weight, slowly, but I was clearly making better choices.

I gave one dog to my son. I put an ad on Craigslist for the other dog, and within hours I was getting calls. I made 500 dollars selling her. It was a tremendous relief.

I had been applying for a number of new jobs, feeling desperate to get out of my job. I had a number of interviews and turn-downs, but one day before I was headed to a tapping training for professionals that the VA was paying for, I was called and told I had gotten a new job!!!

The tapping training was great, and I was already feeling better. I had stopped crying all the time, and I actually was calmer during the training than many of the others in there. I couldn't work up a good negative emotion even though I tried. I did work on some stuff, but it didn't cause me great distress.

I started my new job and it was a breath of fresh air! I was still working out and losing some weight, and also losing inches.

By my daughter's wedding, I had lost 20 pounds, had found a wonderful mother-of-the-bride dress and was looking forward to seeing all the friends and family that were flying in to be at the wedding. I had stopped feeling alone, and took in all the people who spent their time and money to come to the wedding. My friend said, "You know, everyone is here because of you!!!" I began to really get it that I had a lot of people in my life, and although I had lost my immediate family (mother, father, brother and husband). I had more people in my life than most people do. It was a wonderful wedding, full of love and wonderful feelings. I was truly able to take it in, spend time with the many different groups of friends and relatives, and put it out there that I was doing so much better.

I had totally stopped crying in my therapist's office, and I was mostly coming in with great news. I had started working out hard and losing weight and inches. I planned a trip to New York to surprise a friend for her sixtieth birthday, and my friends got together to plan a birthday party for me for my sixtieth! I felt loved.

In addition, I got back into my jewelry business. It doesn't freak me out anymore. It's a great source of extra income, but I don't have to be driven about it.

I found a company that could help me with my loans. Life was starting to feel manageable. I found a condo that was more house than I could ever have imagined I could afford. It was under contract, but the person couldn't qualify for the loan. They prequalified me in minutes!!! I thought the universe had finally changed course!

Recently, a number of social workers were asked if they were interested in a new position at a new clinic. The job would mean a big promotion and raise. Looking at the increase in salary, and with retirement staring me in the face, I decided to put my hat in the ring, knowing that one of my colleagues had been promised this job. One week later, last Thursday, my bosses called me into their office and said, "The job is yours!!!"

So, the tally from tapping has been: Twenty pounds lost (with more to go), working out consistently, two job offers, and now I will be starting a new job, same responsibilities, with more salary. I am living in a brand-new condo. I haven't cried in my therapist's office for a long time. I have a few jewelry parties, all of which came as a result of being asked by former hostesses, rather than my soliciting them. I still have some work to do, but my life has changed in one year of tapping!

Chapter 12
And Finally . . .

When to Use EFT

Use EFT when you feel stressed. You may be surprised at how much better you can feel. But also try it *before* you are stressed – before you give a talk in front of a group, before that family get-together, before you drive on the freeway where you saw the wreck. Don't wait until a problem gets big before you use the tapping – it only takes a minute, but it can make a big difference.

Tap when you are stuck or in a rut. Remember that you can tap for what you want, as well as for what you don't want. Tap for new opportunities, for creative ideas to make your life better.

Tap when you are confused, when you are not sure of which way to go or what to choose. Tap when you need answers and don't know where they will come from.

Tap when you feel overwhelmed, when you are too busy and don't have enough time or energy or money for everything you need to do. Tap when it's all too much and you can't do it all, but don't know what to give up.

Tap if you're in a relationship or a job that is unhealthy, and you don't know how to get out of it. Tap if life is wearing you down, not letting you be the person you really are.

Tap if you've made a mistake and don't know how to fix it, or even if you blame yourself for things that are really not your fault.

Tap if you don't want to take medicine or you can't afford it or it causes side effects for you or you don't want to get dependent. Tap if the medicines don't work or only help a little bit.

But also tap when you feel good. With tapping, you might dream up new ways to be happy. Tap when things are going well – and you may see other ways you can use your talents.

Personal Peace Process

Over a lifetime, we accumulate a long list of events that we don't like, from major disasters to little annoyances. Even the small things add up, and the result is that our energy is sapped by the things in our past. If each problem has even a small effect on you, the total can be a big energy drain. To reduce the effect of these events on our lives, Gary Craig recommends what he calls the personal peace process.

To do this, make a list of everything in your life that happened that wasn't what you wanted, both big events and little annoyances. List things that happened in your life that were problems that you wish had gone differently, that you wish you hadn't done, or that you wish had not happened to you. You may want to take several days to put together your list. Then go through the list and give each event a SUDS.

On the first day, pick an event with a low SUDS and tap on it until you get it to zero. Aim for three events every day, although if one takes a long time to come down, you may want to do only that one event that day. You may want to use the Choices Method – tap for what the annoyance is, and then for what you would prefer.

If you tap for three events every day, that is ninety events in a month that have less power over you, that are not taking away your energy, that are no longer an issue. You will likely notice a change in your energy level, as those old issues have stopped robbing your energy.

Here is what I want:

I want you to have more control over your stress. I want you to have some tools to use when things are bad, or even when they are just annoying.

I want Olga, and all the Olgas, to know how to stay out of the emergency room and be able to live a peaceful, calm life.

I want EFT offered to every veteran.

I want everyone to know about EFT. I don't want it to be a secret any more. You can help by telling your friends and family about it. It doesn't have to be through my book – there are many teachers and therapists, books, and videos. I learned the most from Gary Craig, but also from Carol Look, Margaret Lynch, Nick Ortner, Jessica Ortner, and others.

I wish you peace and happiness – and keep tapping!

Acknowledgements

I want to thank the Veterans Administration, which gave me the opportunity to prove to myself that EFT works for stress. VA supervisors usually didn't know I was doing it, and sometimes didn't approve, but they helped to make this book possible anyway.

Cyndy White, Rachel Bensinger and Joan Collins were willing to co-create a new type of group for veterans. Dr. Patricia Alexander made sure that veterans had access to EFT when that access was threatened.

Thanks to Roger Callahan and Gary Craig for creating/discovering/perfecting this technique. We all owe them. Thanks to Dr. Audrey Hoo for introducing me to it, and thank you to the EFT teachers who were my teachers. There were many, but I particularly want to mention Carol Look, Pat Carrington and Margaret Lynch.

My parents, Malcolm and Roberta Ritchie, were always supportive, and I am grateful for their trust and love.

Thanks to BJ, Megan, Matt, and Jenny for being there when I needed you.

And thanks to Tom Bird for his amazing guidance for authors.

www.ingramcontent.com/pod-product-compliance
Lightning Source LLC
Chambersburg PA
CBHW070025110426
42741CB00034B/2592